BEST 101

TIPS

TO STOP

HAIR LOSS

DON'T GO BALD

By

Charles Young Jr. R.T.(R) (MR) (ARRT)

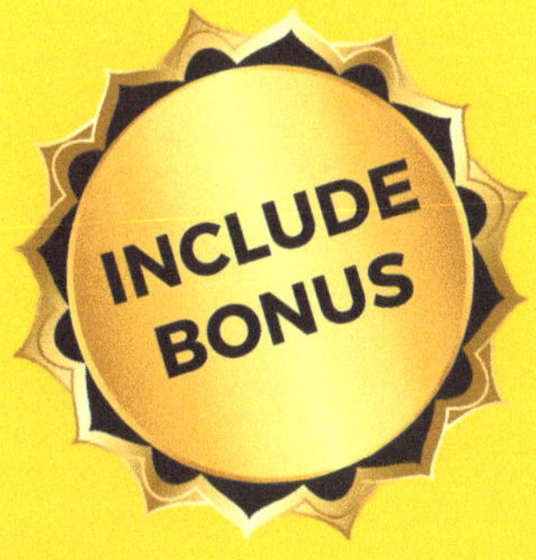

No art of this book may be reproduced in any form or by any electronic or mechanical means, including information storage and retrieval systems, without permission from the author, except for the use of brief quotations in a book review.

ISBN: 978-1-300-84187-6
Imprint: Lulu.com

Published by DFCS Publishing

Disclaimer: The information provided in this book is for educational and informational purposes only. It is not intended to be a substitute for professional medical advice, diagnosis, or treatment. Always seek the advice of your physician or other qualified health provider with any questions you may have regarding a medical condition.

The author and publisher of this book have made every effort to ensure that the information provided is accurate and up-to-date at the time of publication. However, they make no representations or warranties of any kind, express or implied, about the completeness, accuracy, reliability, suitability, or availability of the information contained herein.

The techniques, strategies, and suggestions outlined in this book may not be suitable for every individual. The author and publisher disclaim any responsibility for any adverse effects or consequences resulting from the use or application of the information presented in this book.

Individual results may vary. The success stories and testimonials included in this book are not necessarily indicative of the results you may achieve. Your results may differ due to individual factors, including but not limited to your health condition, genetics, lifestyle, and commitment to following the advice provided.

The mention of specific products, services, organizations, or professionals in this book does not imply endorsement or recommendation by the author or publisher, unless explicitly stated.

By reading this book, you agree to assume full responsibility for your own health and well-being. You acknowledge that the information provided is not a substitute for professional medical advice and that you will consult with a qualified healthcare professional before making any decisions regarding your health or lifestyle.

Best 101 Tips to Stop Hair Loss

Dandruff or scalp psoriasis

When the skin on the scalp is inflamed and itchy, it's obviously tempting to scratch it. But that may cause your hair to shed more than usual.

Dandruff is the most easily treated cause of hair loss because you can treat it with over-the-counter products, like a shampoo containing zinc pyrithione or exfoliating ingredients. "Consistency is the trick," so it's important to find a shampoo and conditioner you like enough to use regularly.

But other conditions can also cause itchiness and scalp flaking, including seborrheic dermatitis (a more severe version of dandruff caused by a buildup of yeast and oil) and psoriasis (an autoimmune condition that causes thick patches of skin). Treating these issues may take more time and effort than dandruff, so it's important to check in with a dermatologist if you think you may be dealing with one of these conditions.

Changes in birth control

Going off hormonal birth control or changing to a different type of hormonal contraception can also cause hormone-induced shedding. "Whether you're just starting it, discontinuing it, or changing brands, your body can react by causing the hair to go into an increased shedding mode."

This is another form of telogen effluvium, which means that it's usually temporary. You can rely on volumizing products and styling tricks while you wait for your hair to regain its fullness.

Intense emotional or physical stress

When you're experiencing something stressful or traumatic—not your average day-to-day stress, but something big and life-altering like a divorce, a death in the family, a significant job change, or a big move—you may experience a temporary halt in hair growth as your body puts its resources toward getting you through said big event.

"Hairs don't all grow at the same rate". "Some are growing, some are resting, and some are actively being shed. When you have these conditions, your body halts hair growth, and then things get restarted and all these hairs that have been halted start to get pushed out at the same time." The same thing can happen with physical stress and trauma, like having a big operation, being hospitalized, or even losing a significant amount of weight very quickly.

Usually, this type of hair shedding is temporary. But if it bothers you, check in with a dermatologist to learn more about styling changes and products you can use to make your hair look and feel fuller.

04 Medications

Some "medications can cause chronic shedding,". In particular, those used to manage high blood pressure, cancer, arthritis, and depression are known to cause hair loss issues.

If you think your medication may be causing hair loss, check in with your doctor. In many cases, this type of hair loss is temporary. But if your hair loss becomes chronic, your doctor may be able to prescribe a different medication that doesn't cause this side effect.

05 Childbirth

Normally, your hair goes through three major life stages. First, there's a growth phase; second, there's a transitional phase when the growing stops but the hair doesn't fall out; and then there's a resting phase. Finally, after the resting phase, your hair falls out.

But during pregnancy, most people notice their hair going into rapid growth mode. "That's when everything is in a grow, grow, grow phase, because there are surges of hormones [estrogen] that make hair grow,". Not only is the growth stage kicked into high gear, but also it lasts longer than normal, meaning that normal shedding doesn't occur.

Once estrogen levels go back to normal after delivery, hair resumes its normal growth cycles and starts to shed all that thick, luscious hair that accumulated over the last 10 months. Some women experience very mild shedding, but others experience intense shedding for a few months.

This type of hair loss (technically, hair shedding) is called telogen effluvium, and it can occur months after a stressful or major life event like childbirth."Shedding peaks about four months after the incident" that caused it.

Postpartum hair loss is, luckily, temporary. So, you don't really have to do anything to treat it, the AAD says. But there are ways to make your hair look and feel fuller while you wait. For instance, look for volumizing shampoos and conditioners that are formulated for fine hair and avoid products that weigh down the hair.

Genetics

When we think of hereditary hair loss, we usually go straight to male pattern baldness. But people of all genders are susceptible to hereditary hair loss. In women the hair loss is usually concentrated at the crown of the head (especially noticeable at the hair part), while it's more likely to affect men along the hairline.

Although you can't prevent this type of hair loss entirely, there are treatments available—such as over-the-counter minoxidil or finasteride—that can slow it down and make hair stay fuller longer. So, the sooner you start treatment, the better. Keep in mind that your treatment options for any condition or health issue on this list may change over time based on new research and newly available therapies. Make sure you have ongoing conversations with your doctor about which treatment options may be best for you.

Overprocessing your hair

Getting frequent perms, chemical straightening procedures, or relaxing procedures—basically anything that uses harsh chemicals on your scalp and hair—can damage the hair follicle and cause permanent hair loss. "After repeated insults, the hair follicles just won't grow back,". This can cause hair to appear thinner and may be especially noticeable on the scalp.

You can prevent further damage by avoiding those harsh procedures and using products designed to help hydrate and heal your hair and scalp. But if you want your hair to grow back, you'll likely need to enlist the guidance of a board-certified dermatologist.

Nutritional deficiencies

Creating and maintaining healthy hair relies on getting solid nutrition. In particular, deficiencies in iron, zinc, vitamin B3 (niacin), and protein have all been linked to various types of hair loss.

Treating a nutritional deficiency usually starts with a chat with your doctor and a blood test to accurately diagnose your issue. Then your doctor may treat your deficiency with prescription supplements or may refer you to an R.D. for further guidance.

Heat-styling your hair regularly

You mayhave something called trichorrhexis nodosa. This is a condition in which damaged, weak points in the hair shaft cause hair to break off easily. The cause? Thermal damage to the hair from things like using hot tools and overbleaching. In this case, the hair loss "is not necessarily from the root but it's from somewhere along the shaft,".

Treatment for trichorrhexis nodosa usually involves finding and avoiding the source of the damage, which could be hot tools, harsh chemicals, or aggressive brushing. Instead, opt for gentle brushing techniques and gentle, soothing hair products.

Autoimmune diseases

"An autoimmune condition makes the body recognize its own hair follicles as foreign and it attacks them and makes the hair fall out,".

This could be a condition like alopecia areata, in which the immune system attacks the hair follicles. Sometimes people with alopecia areata do see their hair grow back (although it may fall out again). But if not, dermatologists can help by prescribing various treatments, like corticosteroid injection to stimulate hair growth.

Conditions that primarily affect another part of the body—like thyroid disease, rheumatoid arthritis, or sickle-cell anemia—can also cause hair loss as one of many symptoms. Additionally, lupus can cause some scarring of the hair follicle, resulting in permanent hair loss.

These conditions can be serious and require an accurate diagnosis from an experienced health care provider. So, if you think your hair loss may be connected to an underlying issue like an autoimmune condition, it's important to talk to your doctor.

Wearing too-tight hairstyles too often

This can cause traction alopecia. "Classically, this happens when people wear tight braids chronically, but I've seen it with tight ponytails too,". It can cause progressive thinning of the hairline, and if you do it for long enough, the hair loss may become permanent. It's considered a scarring process, which can damage the hair follicle beyond repair.

To help prevent and treat hair loss due to traction alopecia, never wear one hairstyle for too long, and try not to pull too tightly if you can help it.

Try leave-on products.

Leave-in conditioners and detanglers help keep your hair moisturized throughout the day and protect against the effects of heat styling that otherwise can cause thinning and breakage.

Wash as often as you need to—but no more.

Both under- and over washing can affect the volume and feel of your hair. Not washing enough causes a buildup of product and oil that can weight your hair down. But washing too frequently can strip the hair of its natural oils, making it drier and more prone to breakage. Try sticking to washing about two or three times per week and adjusting as needed for your particular situation.

Style your hair gently—and without heat, if possible.

Because heat can cause damage to the hair that leads to shedding and breakage, it's important to limit or avoid heat styling entirely. And when putting your hair up, choose styles that don't put too much pressure on your hair or scalp. Styles like tight braids, dreads, and ponytails can be particularly damaging when worn repeatedly or for extended periods of time.

Always use conditioner after shampooing.

Conditioner makes your hair shinier and helps reduce static electricity, both of which helps thinning hair look fuller and glossier. But remember: A little goes a long way, and too much will weigh hair down.

Use hair masks for deep conditioning.

If your hair tends to be dry and brittle, an occasional deep-conditioning mask may be just what it needs to regain some life and strength. These can also help hair look shinier.

Alopecia areata treatment

Treatments for alopecia areata include injecting small amounts of steroids like triamcinolone into affected patches to stimulate hair growth. Although localized injections may not be practical for large areas, often this is a very effective treatment in helping the hairs return sooner. Other treatments, such as oral steroids, other immunosuppressives, or ultraviolet light therapy, are available for more widespread or severe cases but may be impractical for most patients because of potential side effects or risks. In most mild cases, patients can easily cover up or comb over the affected areas.

In more severe and chronic cases, some patients wear hairpieces; nowadays, some men shave their whole scalp now that this look has become fashionable.

Finasteride (Propecia)

This medication is FDA-approved for use in only men with androgenic hair loss. Finasteride is in a class of medications called 5-alpha reductase inhibitors. It helps reduce hair loss by blocking the action of natural hormones in scalp hair follicles. Propecia is a lower-dose version of a commercially available drug called Proscar that helps shrink enlarged prostates in middle-aged and older men. Women of child-bearing potential should avoid finasteride. Propecia 1 mg tablets are available by prescription and taken once daily. Propecia may grow and thicken hair to some extent for some people, but its main use is to keep (maintain) hair that's still there. Studies have shown that this medication works well in some types of hair loss, and patients should use it for about six to 12 months before full effects are determined. This medication does not "work" in days to weeks, and its onset of visible improvement tends to be gradual. It may be best for men who still have enough hair to retain but also can help some regrow hair. Possible but very unlikely side effects include impotence or a decreased sex drive (libido).

Nioxin

Nioxin has been a popular brand of shampoo for hair loss, but there is no compelling evidence showing it is any more effective than regular shampoos. These products are usually harmless but generally not scientifically proven and therefore potentially useless.

Minoxidil (Rogaine)

This topical medication is available over the counter, and no prescription is required. Men and women can use it. It works best on the crown, less on the frontal region. Minoxidil is available as a 2% solution, a 4% solution, an extra-strength 5% solution, and a new foam or mousse preparation. Rogaine may grow a little hair, but it's better at holding onto what's still there. There are few side effects with Rogaine. The main problem with this treatment is the need to keep applying it once or twice daily, and most men get tired of it after a while. In addition, minoxidil tends to work less well on the front of the head, which is where baldness bothers most men. Inadvertent application to the face or neck skin can cause unwanted hair growth in those areas.

Let your hair air-dry

It's the easiest fix you never considered. Hair dryers and irons, especially if your hair is color treated, can cause breakage and thinning, so reduce your use whenever you can.

22 Hormone therapy

Some women are genetically predisposed to female-pattern hair loss or experience increased thinning during menopause, when your estrogen takes a dip. Birth control pills and other forms of hormone replacement therapy, such as estrogen and progesterone pills or creams, can help boost your levels to ward off hair loss.

23 Eat the right nutrients

Again, hair thrives on protein, iron, zinc, omega-3 fatty acids, vitamin A, magnesium, and vitamin B12. To ensure you get the most nutritional bang for your buck, load up on foods that fight hair loss with these nutrients, like lean meats, leafy greens, nuts, beans, sweet potatoes, and fish.

24 Cortisone shots

They hurt, but they can prove effective. Injecting cortisone directly into the scalp blocks the hormonal activity that induces hair thinning. This works especially well in patients with inflammatory scalp disease.

25 Take time to de-stress

Both sudden and chronic stress can halt hair growth. If you've been going through a challenging experience, your hair should grow back once you give your body a break. If you're under constant pressure, consider stress-relieving techniques like meditation.

26 Massage your scalp

You're halfway there every time you shampoo: Massaging your head in the shower can increase blood flow to the scalp. This means a better environment for hair growth, and it also aids the penetration of any treatment shampoos you use.

27 OLLY Hair, Skin & Nails supplements

OLLY Hair, Skin & Nails supplements also contain a blend of biotin, vitamin C, E, and keratin protein to help you fight free radicals that damage hair follicles. You can also take a biotin supplement alone, which helps the body break down fats and carbohydrates to grow stronger strands.

28 Nutrafol

Another hair supplement to consider, "This uses highly concentrated botanicals to address every stage of the growth cycle. It has excellent clinical studies to support its efficacy.

29 Eat More Protein

In order to promote hair growth and healthy hair, your body needs to get enough protein from the foods you eat. If you aren't getting enough protein in your diet, it can disrupt the life cycle of your hair and cause it to begin to fall out within two to three months. Increase the amount of protein you are getting in your diet by eating more meats, eggs, fish, nuts, seeds, and beans.

30 Switch to Products with Gentler Ingredients

In many cases, hair breakage results from using harsh products on your hair. If you frequently bleach your hair or use chemicals to curl or straighten your hair, it can become damaged and look thin. Even everyday synthetic hair products, such as gels and hairsprays, can dry your hair out and cause it to break off. To reduce the risk of hair loss and maintain your healthy hair, limit your use of hair products or ask your hair care professional to recommend some natural products to treat and style your hair.

31 Blood work

Routine blood work can test your ferritin (iron stored in the blood) and vitamin D levels. Low levels can lead to hair loss, and the solution may be as simple eating more iron-rich foods or adding a vitamin D supplement to your routine. Talk to your doctor about the appropriate dosage.

32 Get Regular Trims

When hair loss occurs because your hair is damaged and prone to breakage, regular haircuts can help it look better. Hair that is regularly trimmed is less likely to become damaged and develop brittle split ends, which can travel up your hair shaft toward your scalp. So, although it may sound contrary to your goal if you're trying to grow your hair, regular haircuts may actually help you with hair growth, as they may help keep your hair healthy and prevent it from breaking off.

Shampoo Less

When many people shampoo their hair, they feel as if they are taking good care of it. But daily or repetitive shampooing can actually damage your hair, cause it to easily break, and leave it looking thin. This is because wet hair is more elastic than dry hair and more prone to breakage when you are scrubbing it. To preserve the thickness and health of your hair and prevent hair loss, shampoo less often.

Take Biotin Supplements

Biotin is a B vitamin that is sometimes used to help reduce or prevent hair loss. Some people do not get enough biotin in their diet, resulting in biotin deficiency. Taking biotin supplements may help alleviate hair thinning if you have a biotin deficiency. Talk with your doctor if you suspect that you are deficient in biotin. He can assess your symptoms and determine whether biotin supplements may help you.

Other Autoimmune Diseases

Alopecia areata is just one of many types of autoimmune diseases that can cause hair loss. Hashimoto's thyroiditis and lupus are two examples of other autoimmune diseases that can result in hair loss. This type of hair loss may not always be reversible — it may sometimes be permanent. But medications and hair restoration surgeries may help compensate for any hair loss.

When you have one autoimmune disease, you're at risk for developing others. This is why it's especially important for your doctor to monitor you carefully for any new symptoms or other changes.

Thyroid Problems

Other types of hormone-related conditions may also contribute to hair loss. Some may involve thyroid hormones. Either an underactive thyroid (a medical condition called hypothyroidism), or an overactive thyroid (hyperthyroidism), can result in hair loss because each condition causes a hormonal imbalance. Autoimmune diseases of the thyroid gland, such as Hashimoto's thyroiditis and Graves' disease may also contribute to hair loss.

Thyroid hormones help regulate nearly every function in the body, including hair growth. The right treatment to control either of these thyroid conditions will get hormones under control, stop hair loss, and allow your hair to starting grow back.

Hormonal Imbalances

"Excess androgens, or male sex hormones, and hormonal imbalances are the most common cause of hair loss such as androgenetic alopecia,". Androgens play a role in female and male pattern baldness. In female-pattern baldness, androgens can cause weak hair follicles, also leading to excess shedding. Androgen sensitivities may be exacerbated during estrogen-related changes, such as birth control use or menopause.

Male pattern baldness, on the other hand, is related to an increase in an androgen called dihydrotestosterone (DHT). DHT not only binds to hair follicles and stops hair growth, but it may also decrease a hair's life span overall. This is also called androgenetic alopecia. There are a number of additional medical conditions that may cause this type of hair loss. These include high blood pressure, heart disease, prostate cancer, and polycystic ovary syndrome (PCOS).

Pregnancy

Other hormonal imbalances can also lead to hair loss, especially the wildly fluctuating hormones that happen following pregnancy and childbirth. "Postpartum hair loss is common and affects 40 to 50 percent of women who have recently given birth,". Estrogen levels skyrocket during pregnancy, which can temporarily alter your hair growth cycles. During this time, you're likely to experience less hair loss than normal.

As estrogen levels return to normal after pregnancy, you may notice more hair loss than usual. It's also not uncommon for postpartum moms to notice thinning hair or even patches of baldness. Postpartum hair loss may happen one to six months after childbirth, with symptoms lasting up to 18 months. "Because not all hair follicles in the resting stage during pregnancy will move into the shedding phase at once, excessive shedding can last 6 to 15 months postpartum,". Postpartum related hair loss is most noticeable along the hairline, as well as in women with long hair. As the rest of your body recovers, so will your hair follicles. The hair loss is only temporary — your hair will grow back. While postpartum hair loss isn't exactly preventable, you can minimize the problem by taking it easy on your hair and keeping up with your prenatal vitamins.

39 Trichotillomania

While stress is often a short-term cause of hair loss, severe stress or anxiety may be associated with hair-pulling disorder, or trichotillomania. Mental health condition is related to obsessive-compulsive disorder and other types of anxiety disorders. Aside from compulsive hair pulling, other signs of trichotillomania include feeling relief or pleasure after hairs are pulled, as well noticeable patches of hair loss. Trichotillomania most often develops between ages 10 and 13, but it's considered a chronic problem that may improve with treatment.

Also, if you're dealing with hair loss from other causes and have a history of hair-pulling disorders, it's possible to experience trichotillomania as a stress response. If you suspect you may have this mental health condition, there are treatments that can help, such as cognitive behavioral therapy and habit reversal training. These types of therapies can help you be more cognizant of urges to pull your hair, and help you develop other coping mechanisms instead. Additionally, while no medications are approved for trichotillomania alone, certain antidepressants or antipsychotics may help.

40 Extreme Hair Care

In an effort to create a stylish hairdo, you can actually cause significant damage and breakage, which could result in hair loss and thinning hair. Shampooing or blow-drying too frequently, repeatedly using heated styling tools, pulling on hair — whether while blow-drying it or styling it in a too-tight ponytail, for instance — or too vigorously rubbing the scalp can all lead to hair loss. Perms, relaxers, and hair dyes may also contribute to damage-induced hair loss. "Seek out shampoos and conditioners that are mild and suited for your hair to avoid unnecessary damage".

41 Physical Trauma

When your body is under serious physical stress, the natural cycle of hair growth and rest can be disrupted, resulting in hair loss, often in the form of thinning hair — your hair may even come out in clumps. Any shock to the system, such as a severe accident, surgery, burns, or serious illness, can also shock the hair follicles. This may result in up to 50 to 75 percent of your hair falling out, sometimes months after the fact. This type of hair loss is also known as telogen effluvium, and it may resolve within six to eight months.

Infections and illnesses can also lead to hair loss. A high fever or a severe infection can all contribute to temporary hair loss. These physical traumas may include fungal skin infections, as well as bacterial infections like syphilis, which can all be responsible for balding or thinning hair. Treatment of the underlying infection can restore hair growth and prevent future hair loss, so your first step is to seek medical attention for the primary health problem.

 ## Certain Medications

Hair loss is a side effect of a number of medications taken for common health problems. This is also known as "drug-induced hair loss." Blood-thinning medications, oral contraceptives, drugs for depression, anti-inflammatories, and beta and calcium channel blockers can all lead to thinning hair or baldness. Too much vitamin A and vitamin A–based drugs called retinoids can cause hair loss as well. Some chemotherapy drugs used to treat cancer are known to cause total hair loss as they work to destroy cancer cells. Just as hair usually grows back after chemo, it should also grow back once you stop taking any medication that causes hair loss. But don't stop taking prescribed medications without talking to a doctor first — he or she may instead shift you to a different drug to see if hair loss improves.

 ## Hair Regrowth Serums

Many popular and name-brand serums seek to address hair loss or thinning for hair on other parts of the body. These various serums claim to improve eyelash length and thickness and help regrow eyebrow hair — but talk to your doctor before trying them for alopecia-related hair loss. "Using any product near the eyes carries risk,". "Physician-prescribed bimatoprost solution for use in these delicate areas is advised."

 ## Hair Implants

While it can be tempting to many, be very cautious seeking out implant treatments for alopecia. "Implanted hair that isn't done through a transplant is not an FDA [U.S. Food and Drug Administration] approved treatment,". "Most claims made for hair regrowth are false. The only studies showing over-the-counter improvement in growth that have significant scientific support involve the use of minoxidil."

 ## Get a Professional Hair and Scalp Analysis

Sometimes, it can be difficult to determine why your hair is falling out — and therefore, how to treat or prevent hair loss. In addition to reviewing your medical history and asking about lifestyle factors that may be affecting the health of your hair, a dermatologist can perform a professional hair and scalp analysis to help determine the cause of your hair loss. Your dermatologist will carefully study your hair and scalp and may take a sample of your hair or a scalp biopsy to gather more information.

Change Your Hairstyle

Certain hair accessories — including hairpins, clips, and rubber bands — can cause extensive hair breakage when they are used to hold your hair tightly in place. Tight ponytails, cornrows, or braids can also create tension on your hair and cause it to break and appear thin. Minimizing the use of hair accessories and not continuously wearing hairstyles that pull on your hair. And when you do use hair accessories, select hairpins with balled ends, clips with rubber padding, and fabric hair ties instead of rubber bands.

Limit Brushing for Healthy Hair

Vigorous grooming of your hair — such as following the old recommendation to brush it 100 strokes every night — can damage your hair and cause it to break off. If you excessively brush your hair and it appears thin or shaggy, try limiting how much you brush your hair. Often, the best way to improve the health of your hair is to leave it alone as much as possible.

Consume More Iron

If your diet doesn't include enough iron, it could cause your hair to fall out. Your doctor can check this with a blood test. If you are iron deficient, an easy fix to help prevent hair loss is to increase the amount of dietary iron you consume. Good sources of iron include organ meats, clams, oysters, iron-fortified cereals, beans, pumpkin seeds, and spinach. But don't take an iron supplement without talking with your doctor — too much iron can be harmful.

Use a hard Water Softener to control hair fall

After getting the water quality tested, if you find out that you get hard water, it's time to install a water softener to prevent hair fall. The only way to deal with the hard water problem and save your hair from excessive damage is by using soft water. The traditional methods of softening water don't serve your purpose and are time-taking. A water softener automatically converts hard water into soft. The non-electric appliance exchanges excessive minerals such as calcium and magnesium with sodium, thereby making the water soft. The compact size makes it easy to install the softener even if you have space constraints. The effective hair fall solution will improve your tresses to a great extent and also prevent breakage.

Quick Tip: Install a bathroom water softener to get a continuous supply of soft water

Regular Oil Massage

Oiling your hair has a lot of benefits. Make sure you mix essential oils such as lavender, castor, and almond oils. Massage your scalp at least for 15 minutes. Massaging your scalp improves blood circulation, thereby reducing the chances of hair loss.

Exercise

Exercising is the key to good hair. Depending on your preference, you can swim, walk or hit the gym for at least 30 minutes a day to balance the hormone levels, reduce stress, and improve blood circulation to reduce hair loss.

Keep your Scalp Sweat-Free

Oily hair leads to dandruff, especially during summer as a result of sweating. This also increases the chances of hair fall. Keep your scalp sweat-free and clean by using a mild shampoo. You can use shampoos that have neem to keep your scalp clean and dandruff-free.

Use a Mild Shampoo

Instead of using shampoos loaded with chemicals, go for natural and herbal shampoos. Regularly washing your hair with mild shampoo keeps your scalp clean, thereby reducing the risk of infections and dandruff. When your scalp is clean, it reduces the chances of hair loss.

Protect your Hair from Sun

The harmful sun rays cause a lot of damage to your hair. The harsh sun rays make your hair shaft brittle and dry, leading to hair fall. Make sure you cover your hair when you go out to save your hair from sun damage.

Quick Tip: Use a hat or leave-in conditioner to avoid damage

Tie your Hair when Sleeping

This tip is handy for people with long or medium-length hair. Make sure you tie your hair when sleeping to prevent your hair from being tangled or frizzy. This will prevent hair breakage and hair loss.

Use Garlic, Onion, or Ginger Juice

To avoid hair fall, rub garlic, onion, or ginger juice on your scalp. Leave it overnight and wash it in the morning. Make sure to follow this routine once a week for noticeable results.

Stay Away from Chemical Treatments

Hair coloring, or straightening your hair has a negative effect on your hair. If you are already suffering from hair loss, make sure you don't undergo any type of chemical treatment as it may worsen the situation.

Avoid Hot Water Bath

Hair is very delicate, so it is important to avoid excessively hot water to wash your hair. Hot water steals away color and activates the oil-producing glands. Use lukewarm water to dilute the secretion of oil glands and improve blood circulation.

Rub Green Tea

Green tea is not only good for weight loss but also keeps your hair healthy. Rubbing green tea into hair may curb hair loss problems. Brew two tea bags of green tea in a cup of water and leave it to cool. Apply it to your hair to rinse thoroughly.

Get Sufficient Sleep

Lack of sleep affects your hair and skin. Make sure you get at least 7-8 hours of sleep on a daily basis, which will solve many of your hair problems.

Use Homemade Hair Masks

Homemade hair masks are a great way to keep your hair healthy and prevent breakage. Use homemade hair masks made from onion, beetroot, green tea, neem leaves, and fruits to maintain your hair healthy and prevent breakage.

Don't Rub your Hair

Many people make the mistake of rubbing their hair right after taking a bath. This habit not only makes your hair dry but also increases the chances of hair loss and breakage. Make sure you don't rub your hair with a dry towel and let your hair dry naturally.

Avoid Smoking

Smoking not just affects your health but also leads to hair loss. Cigarettes reduce the amount of blood that flows to your scalp, thereby affecting hair growth.

Stay Hydrated

One-quarter of the hair shaft contains water, which is why it is essential to drink a lot of water to avoid hair loss. Make sure you drink at least 3 liters of water per day to stay hydrated and keep your hair healthy.

Don't Brush Wet Hair

Your hair is fragile when it's wet. Combing wet hair increases the chances of hair loss. However, if you must comb wet hair, use a wide-toothed comb to avoid breakage. In addition, don't brush your hair too frequently as it can injure hair and increase hair loss.

Quick Tip: Use a wooden, wide-toothed comb to reduce hair breakage

Include more Protein in your Diet

Lack of protein is also a reason for hair loss. This is the reason why you need to include a lot of protein in your diet if you have a hair fall problem. Eat a lot of lean meat, fish, soy, and other forms of proteins to reduce hair loss and promote hair growth.

Follow a Proper Diet

In addition to the water quality, it is extremely important to follow a healthy diet. Make sure you include important vitamins, and proteins in your diet to avoid hair fall. Eat foods that are loaded with proteins, vitamin E, iron, biotin, and zinc. Foods rich in Vitamin A promote the production of sebum, whereas Vitamin E improves blood circulation and keeps the hair follicles productive. Lean meat, soy, and fish encourage hair health and also curb hair loss. The food items also help in hair growth in addition to maintaining their texture and quality.

Check your Water Quality

One of the common causes of hair loss that most of you oversee is the quality of water. Hard water can cause irreversible damage to your hair. The excessive amount of calcium, magnesium, and salts present in hard water form a layer on your hair strands, which dries out your hair. When your hair is not washed properly, the residue accumulates on your scalp leading to dandruff and breakage. Hard water also has a high pH level, which charges your hair negatively resulting in friction and breakage. Hard water has a pH level of 8.5 whereas the pH level of your hair is 3.5. As the pH level of water is almost 50% higher than the pH of your hair, it damages your tresses. So, if you are losing hair even after using the right products or eating right, the problem lies in your water. The only way to know whether you get hard water is by getting the water quality tested.

Stressful life events

Out of nowhere, you notice a lot of hair falling out. You see it on your pillow, on the floor, on your clothes, and stuck in the shower drain. Hair seems to come out so easily that you may be afraid to brush it. The medical term for this is "telogen effluvium."

During telogen effluvium, it might feel like you're going to go bald. Rest assured — this won't happen. Telogen effluvium is a response to stress. Excess hair shedding starts 2 to 3 months after a stressful physical or emotional event and peaks about 4 to 5 months later. Over time, the body readjusts and hair gradually stops falling out. Within 6 to 9 months, things go back to normal.

Stressful life events, like losing a loved one, going through surgery, or being diagnosed with a serious illness, can all increase the risk for hair loss. But hair loss itself can be stressful, which can lead to a vicious cycle. Most cases of telogen effluvium are temporary and don't require treatment.

Hormonal changes

People with conditions like polycystic ovary syndrome (PCOS) and congenital adrenal hyperplasia (CAH) have higher androgen levels, which can cause female-pattern hair loss. You may want to ask your healthcare provider about having your hormone levels tested if you're a woman who experiences more obvious hair loss and any of these symptoms:

- Acne
- Excess hair growth on the face or body
- Irregular periods
- Other things that can cause dramatic changes in hormone levels — like pregnancy, childbirth, menopause, and hypothyroidism — may also affect hair growth. Even changing medication routines can cause your hair to thin if your medications affect your hormone levels. For example, some women who stop taking birth control pills can experience hair loss. Fortunately, in most of these cases, you can slow down or reverse the hair loss with proper treatment.

71 Infections

Infections can affect the scalp and cause hair to fall out. This happens when bacteria, yeast, or fungi overgrow and invade hair follicles. You might see pus bumps, redness, and scaling. The scalp can feel itchy or even painful. If you notice any of these symptoms, see your dermatologist right away. Fungal infections of the scalp are highly contagious, and they're the most common cause of hair loss in children. To prevent it, children should avoid sharing hats and scarves. Most scalp infections are curable with the right antibiotic or antifungal medication. Without treatment, these infections can lead to permanent scarring.

72 Chemotherapy and radiation

Hair loss can be a very real fear for many people who have received a diagnosis of cancer and need chemotherapy or radiation. Chemotherapy drugs kill cells in the body that grow quickly so that they don't form tumors or spread. But, because cells in hair follicles also grow quickly, chemotherapy can also affect hair.

Radiation therapy, another cancer treatment, can also cause hair loss. But while chemotherapy can cause hair loss throughout the body, radiation therapy usually only affects the area that's treated. With both types of treatments, hair loss is generally temporary. So, you can expect your hair to regrow a few months after the end of treatment.

73 Age

Almost everyone will notice hair loss and hair thinning as they age. Cells continually grow and die off at all ages. But with age, cells die off more quickly than they regenerate. This is why people get weaker bones and thinner skin. And it's a similar process for hair. As you age, you also produce less oil in your scalp, which can make hair weak and brittle. This can also contribute to overall hair loss and thinning. Some people may experience more severe hair loss as they age. This condition is androgenetic alopecia, which is also called female- or male-pattern hair loss. We'll talk more about that below.

74 Traumatic hairstyling

Some hairstyling practices can cause this type of scarring hair loss. If they're not stopped early, they can cause significant hair loss that can't be regrown. Examples of these practices include:

- Heat styling
- Chemical hair treatments
- Tight hairstyles
- Some shampoos that contain the chemical formaldehyde have been linked to hair loss, too. If you notice hair loss after starting a new shampoo, stop using it and try a different product after making sure it doesn't have any formaldehyde in it.

Take supplements

Lack of vitamins in your diet can cause your hair to fall. Taking multivitamin supplements provides a boost of nourishment to your body which can help you reduce hair fall. However, we strongly suggest that you include such supplements in your daily routine only after consulting your doctor.

Avoid chemical or heating products

Heating products and chemical can damage your hair severely. If you are facing hair fall issues, take a break from using any chemical or heating tools on your hair. Believe it or not, this is the best thing that you can do for your hair health.

Try some tried and tested home remedies

You don't always need a salon when you have the option of trying out home remedies to fix your hair woes. A hot oil massage, for example, is not just soothing but effective when it comes to strengthening your hair. The warm oil not only increases the blood circulation but also penetrates deeper into the pores, nourishing your hair and scalp.

Be gentle with your hair

Avoid aggressively drying your hair with a towel. When your hair is wet, it is more prone to breakage. Hence, being gentle is advisable if you want to keep your hair healthy. Also, be gentle while combing your hair. Using a wide-tooth comb while detangling will result in lesser breakage.

Go for ayurvedic treatments

Ayurveda has the answer to all your hair woes including hair fall. Using bhringraj oil or triphala can prove to be very beneficial when it comes to treating hair fall. Triphala is rich in vitamin C and antioxidants which make the hair healthy and reduce the risk of hair breakage. Bhringraj oil, on the other hand, reduces hair loss and stimulates hair growth.

Improve your diet

A proper diet is essential for your overall health, especially your hair health. A diet rich in vitamin C, D, B, E, zinc, iron,omega-3 fatty acids, and proteins can give your hair the nourishment it needs. With proper nourishment, there's less hair damage and hair breakage. Consume foods like eggs, yoghurt, and broccoli which are rich in biotin and protein to make your tresses strong.

Give yoga a try

If the reasons behind your hair fall include lifestyle changes or hormonal issues, yoga can be extremely beneficial. Yoga will help you manage stress and prove to be effective in maintaining hormonal balance. When these underlying issues are resolved, your hair health will also be restored. Certain yoga poses also increase the blood flow to your scalp, promoting hair growth.

Take care of your hair while sleeping

Try braiding your hair before sleeping. This will reduce the damage caused by friction due to the contact between your hair and the pillow. You should also switch your cotton pillowcase to a silk one to reduce your hair fall.

So, reducing hair fall is possible as long as you're ready to make these simple changes to your lifestyle. However, we do recommend that you see a doctor to rule out any underlying medical conditions.

Maintain good scalp hygiene

Just because coronavirus has ensured we stay locked up in our homes doesn't mean it is alright to skip shampooing. You should be washing your hair every once or twice a week. Shampoo prevents extra scalp buildup which can clog your hair follicles, causing hair fall. Remember, overwashing is also not advisable because it can strip your scalp of its natural oils that are essential for healthy hair growth.

Ginseng

Ginseng contains certain phytochemicals that may promote hair growth on the scalp. Further study is needed to recommend specific dosages. In the meantime, speak with your doctor before adding ginseng supplements to your diet.

Hair processing

Chemical treatments, like perms or hair color, may also damage hair and scalp. Ask your stylist about alternatives, like organic hair dyes and others that don't contain ammonia, peroxide, or para-phenylenediamine (PPD).

86 Platelet-rich plasma

Injecting platelet-rich plasma (PRP) into the scalp helps stimulate growth in areas already impacted by hair loss. Blood is run through a centrifuge to separate out the platelets and then injected into the scalp.

Pricing ranges from $1,500 to $3,500 for your first three treatments, and it's unlikely to be covered by insurance.

87 Coconut oil

Coconut oil may help prevent hair damage from grooming and ultraviolet (UV) light exposure. Lauric acid found in coconut oil helps bind in hair, protecting it from breakage at the root and strand. Massaging coconut oil into the scalp may promote better blood flow and help with regrowth.

88 Saw palmetto

Derived from the fruit of American dwarf pine trees, this herb may help men maintain levels of testosterone. Saw palmetto doses of 100–320 mg could help hair quality, hair count, and hair density. Saw palmetto may help people with AGA, telogen effluvium, and self-perceived hair thinning.

89 Mediterranean diet

A diet containing raw vegetables and fresh herbs, like the Mediterranean diet, may reduce the risk of androgenic alopecia (female pattern baldness or male pattern baldness) or slow its onset. For the best results consume high amounts of these foods — like parsley, basil, and salad greens — more than 3 days a week.

90 Onion juice

People with alopecia areata may see regrowth after applying crude onion juice to their scalps twice a day. The juice appear to promote growth. Scientists believe that hair-growing properties may have to do with the onion's sulfur content.

 ## 91 Phenylephrine

Topical phenylephrine may help with hair loss due to styling by stimulating the follicle muscles to contract. This makes it harder to pull out hairs during brushing, for example. Unfortunately, topical phenylephrine isn't publicly available yet.

 ## 92 Laser therapy

Low-level lasers may help improve hair density for people with genetic hair loss and loss due to chemotherapy. This option is also called red light therapy, and it may work by stimulating epidermal stem cells. You can find home laser devices on the market. And you may need to use the device regularly to see results.

 ## 93 Olive oil

Olive oil can be used to deep condition hair, protecting it from dryness and associated breakage. Olive oil is also a central ingredient in the Mediterranean diet, which may help slow genetic hair loss. Consider applying a couple of tablespoons of olive oil directly to the hair and letting it sit for 30 minutes before washing it out.

 ## 94 Regular washing

Washing your hair daily may protect against hair loss by keeping the scalp healthy and clean. The key is to use mild shampoo. Harsher formulas may dry hair and cause it to break, leading to hair loss.

 ## 95 Essential oils

Essential oils may help reduce hair loss. Various essential oils, including chamomile oil, thyme oil, tea tree oil, and others, could improve conditions like alopecia areata, androgenetic alopecia, and psoriatic alopecia.

Other essential oils to consider include lavender, lemongrass, and peppermint. Try mixing couple drops of any or all of these oils with a couple of tablespoons of carrier oil, like jojoba or grapeseed. Apply to the scalp for 10 minutes before washing. But make sure to test any essential oils before trying the above. It's possible to be allergic to essential oils.

Vitamin A

Vitamin A is partly made up of retinoids, which support healthy hair growth and influence the hair cycle. But it's dose-dependent, meaning that too much — or too little — can damage your hair. It's unlikely you'll receive too much vitamin A from dietary sources. So, fill your plate with foods rich in vitamin A, like sweet potatoes, sweet peppers, and spinach, to name a few.

Aloe Vera

Another natural ingredient that helps when dealing with hair fall is Aloe vera. It contains enzymes, which repair dead skin cells on the scalp, promoting healthier hair. Aloe vera also conditions and improves your hair's elasticity, preventing further hair loss when applied directly to the scalp. You can directly apply aloe vera gel to your scalp and let it sit for an hour. Rinse the gel off by proceeding with your normal hair care routine and enjoy your moisturized and hydrated hair.

Fish oil

Fish oil is a known tonics that help boost immunity, overall health, and have positive effects on hair growth too. Omega-3 found in fish oils has properties that help in opening up the hair follicles and promotes blood circulation in the scalp. This keeps the hair and scalp healthy and prevents excessive hair fall. Fish oils are supplements commonly consumed in the form of capsules.

Use A Wooden Comb

After your hair is dry, use a wooden wide-toothed comb to gently detangle any tangles and prevent hair from falling due to static electricity that is common in plastic combs. Also, avoid brushing wet hair as the hair roots are soft and delicate, and your hair can be easily pulled out. Comb from down-up if you have tangles.

100 Indulge In A Hair Spa At Home

If you want to maintain luscious and healthy hair, a hair spa works best. The good news is you can do it at home by following these easy steps:

Step 1: Shampoo your hair.
Step 2: Apply a deep conditioning hair mask.
Step 3: Apply steam to your hair. You can dip a towel in hot water, squeeze the excess water, and wrap the towel around your head. You can also use one of these good hair steamers.
Step 4: Wash off the conditioner. Towel dry.
Step 5: Apply a light oil or serum.

A hair spa at home will make your hair and scalp healthier, the roots stronger, and improve blood circulation. It reduces hair fall and stimulates hair growth by nourishing the hair follicles and removing impurities. Your hair will feel softer and look shinier.

101 Veggies

Vegetables like spinach, raw papaya, bottle gourd, carrot, ladies finger, sweet potato, squash, tomato, beans, and pumpkin are great sources of vitamins and minerals. They help nourish the follicles and make the hair strands stronger. Consume at least 3 different veggies per day in curries or salads.

BONUS

Stay positive and manage stress

Maintaining a positive mindset and effectively managing stress can contribute to overall well-being, which in turn may positively impact hair health. High stress levels can sometimes exacerbate hair loss, so practicing relaxation techniques and engaging in activities you enjoy can make a difference.

For more great eBooks, please visit.

www.best101tips.net